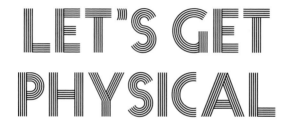

LET'S GET
PHYSICAL

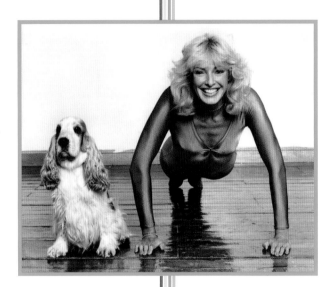

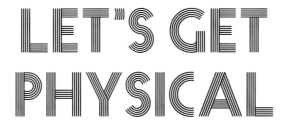

LET'S GET PHYSICAL

Get fit and fabulous the '80s way

Ashley Davies

HarperCollins*Publishers*

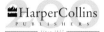

HarperCollins*Publishers*
1 London Bridge Street
London SE1 9GF
www.harpercollins.co.uk

First published by HarperCollins*Publishers* in 2017

10 9 8 7 6 5 4 3 2 1

Copyright © HarperCollins*Publishers* 2017
Text by Ashley Davies
Picture research by Katie Horwich
Design by Gareth Butterworth

Cover image © Universal Images Group
North America LLC / Alamy Stock Photo
Back cover photographs © Shutterstock.com
For full photography credits, see pages 120–125

A catalogue record for this book is available from the British Library

ISBN 978-0-00-827783-3

Printed and bound in Latvia

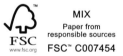

MIX
Paper from
responsible sources
FSC™ C007454

This book is produced from independently certified FSC™ paper
to ensure responsible forest management.

For more information visit: www.harpercollins.co.uk/green

CONTENTS

INTRODUCTION

Providing you were young, energetic and blissfully ignorant about the dangerously selfish socio-economic philosophies of the period, there was a lot of fun to be had in the '80s.

People started realising that exercise didn't just help you look better – it made you feel fantastic too. And, in the true spirit of the time, working out became competitive. That extended to what kind of exercise you did, where you did it, whose programme you followed and, most importantly for a lot of people, how you looked while you were feeling that burn.

In an era of gigantic hair and shoulder pads, brightly coloured outfits and for-God's-sake-please-notice-me accessories, there wasn't an ice-pop's chance in hell that workout wear was going to be drab or humble, and a thriving industry was born. Leg warmers were as huge as the lower half of leotards were tiny.

Crucially, everyone involved was enthusiastic, and that was infectious. So, if you find working out all a bit gloomy these days, perhaps it's time to get physical like they did in the '80s.

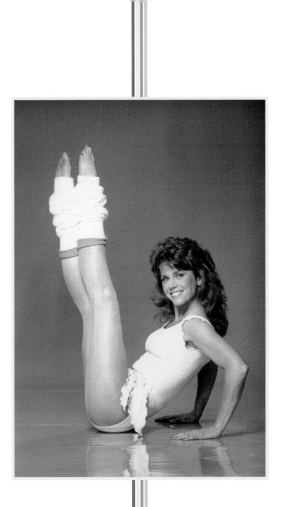

WORK IT

Are the increasingly complicated demands of today's clean-living lifestyle trends getting you down? Is the po-faced approach to wellness starting to feel like a joyless arms race? Do you yearn to inject some genuine happiness into your fitness regime?

There is an alternative. Exercise like it's the '80s and you will feel alive in ways you never dreamt possible. True, mild static electric shocks will be inevitable, but, boy, it will be worth it.

All you need is a bouncy attitude and a willingness to accessorise like your life depends on it. Embellishment is the name of this game. Go big or go home. Here's how to get started.

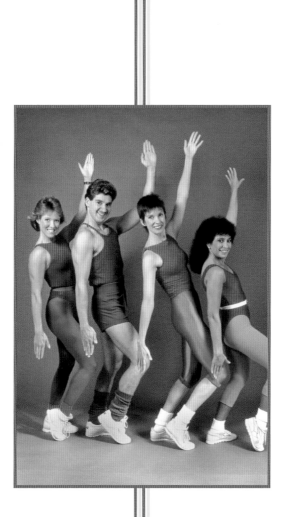

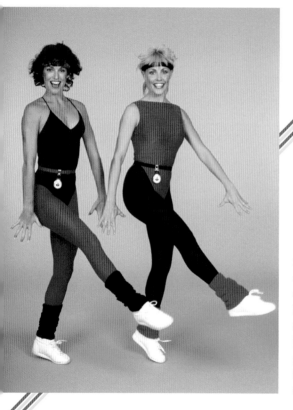

Start by choosing a gym buddy and co-ordinate your outfits. Try to outdo each other's makeup and accessories. If she gets a belt, you get a belt and a headband. If she gets a headband and new leg warmers, put a key ring on your belt. This friendly competition is time-consuming but very motivating.

The road to corporeal perfection is littered with the bodies of rivals. Stay focused. Disguise the painful fury of your ambition with stage makeup.

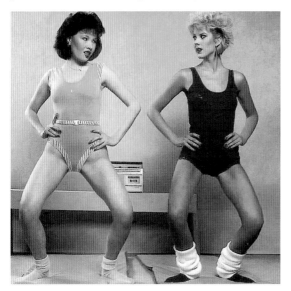

Teamwork is vital though. Take care of your squad and they'll take care of you. A dainty dab of wet-look gel will keep your 'do fresh.

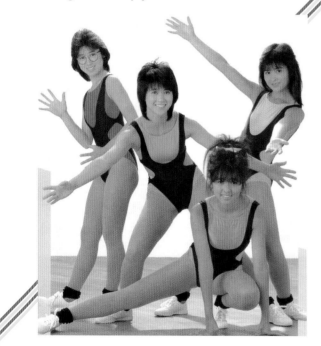

Leg warmers are the beating heart of '80s workout gear. Fight the urge to ask what the actual heck they're for and embrace them. Treasure them. They will prove you're taking this seriously.

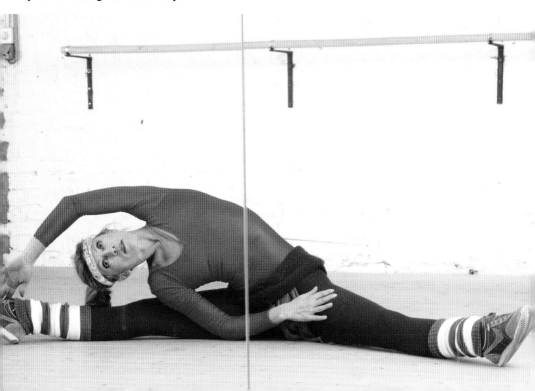

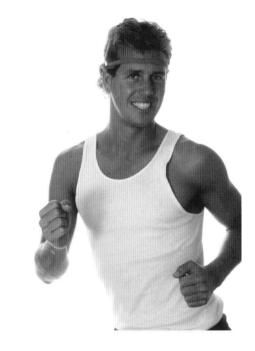

If you're on a budget, simply tie a shoelace around your head and smile convincingly.

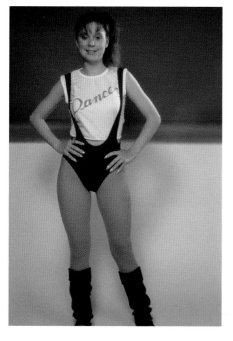

Declaring your preferred method
of artistic expression in diagonal
letters on your shirt will help people
know you are not to be trifled with.

The trend for eye-wateringly high-cut leotard thighs raged unchecked. They got so high that some people struggled to stand up.

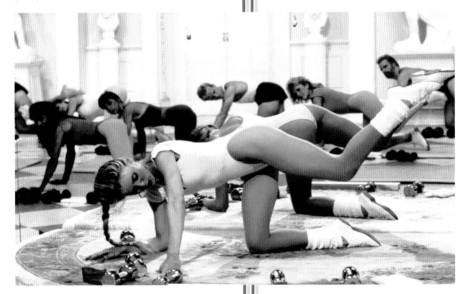

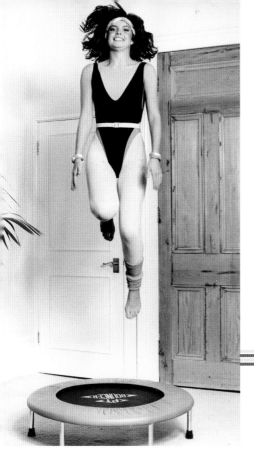

And when they couldn't get any higher, the competitive spirit propelled them upwards in ever-more creative ways.

17

Word to the wise: if you try to disguise your big old socks as leg warmers, you're gonna get the side-eye, big time.

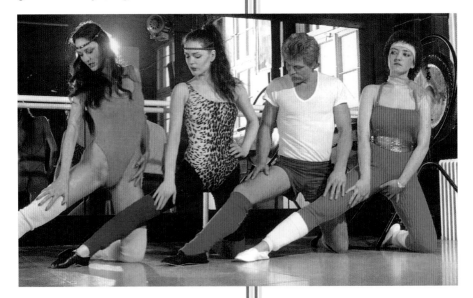

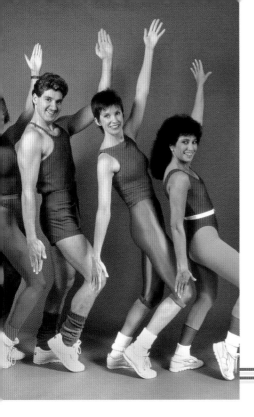

Fellas, you only need to follow
three simple rules if you want
to be accepted: co-ordinate,
co-ordinate, co-ordinate.

If your house burns down or jealous haters steal your leg warmers, get your hands on something bright to stand out at aerobics, ideally a colour blend reminiscent of a toxic hazard warning. Be strong. Be seen. Be safe.

When co-ordinating workout gear with your best friends, select an outfit that represents all three personality types: confident, curious and weak with hunger.

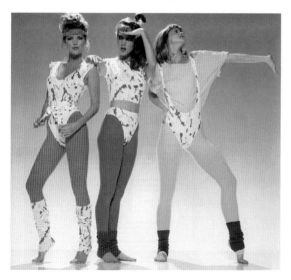

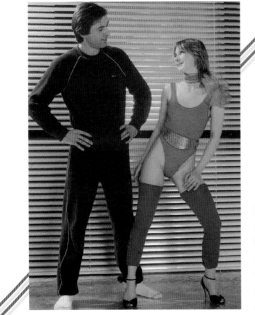

Don't be discouraged if your leotard shrank in the wash and that piece of trash Pam stole your dance shoes: distract pyjama-wearing onlookers with stilettos, a jaunty scarf, a belt made from Christmas crackers and a sassy posture.

If a fully clothed dude approaches you in the gym to mansplain the weights system, what's the first question you ask yourself? That's right. It's: 'Does my ribbon match my gigantic workout earrings?' You're good to go, babez.

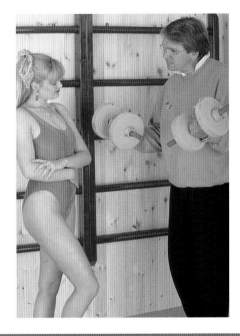

Having hair as big as your dreams is a crucial part of embracing the true joy of '80s fitness culture. True, the amount of hairspray this requires will ruin the ozone layer for future generations, but your frequent flicking motions will result in a fan-like effect to cool your friends down.

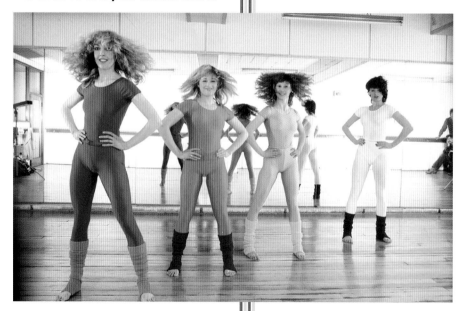

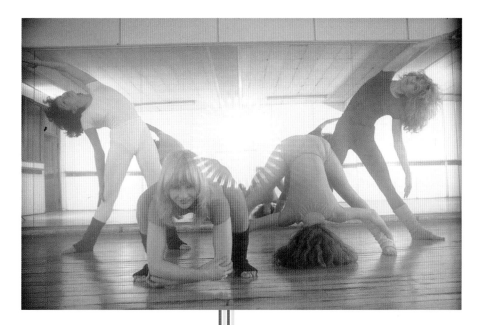

Working out is sweaty business. Take it in turns using your hair to mop up wet patches.

If enormous hair proves to be too hot for comfort, just trim down the area around your face: gym business at the front, party at the back!

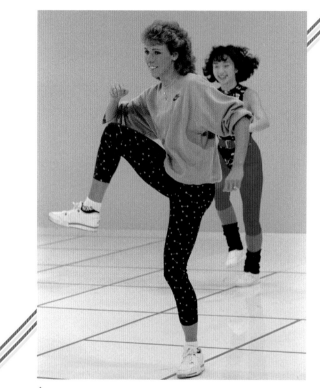

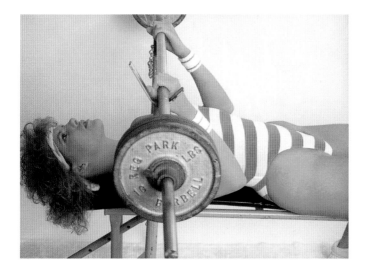

Avoid being seen in unflattering horizontal stripes by simply doing all your exercise lying down.

Hate following the crowd? Embrace your outsider status and wear jeans to the gym. So what if the sheeple turn their backs on you? Their loss.

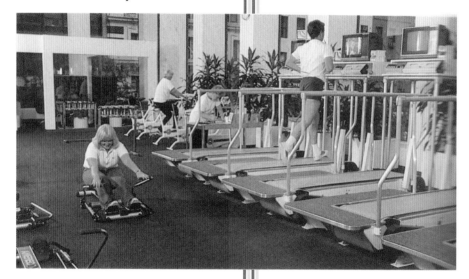

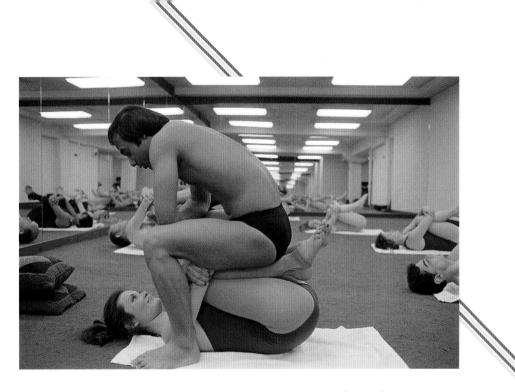

The importance of stretching cannot be understated. In the '80s, a man in Speedos would go from gym to gym, sitting on ladies in the name of hamstring health.

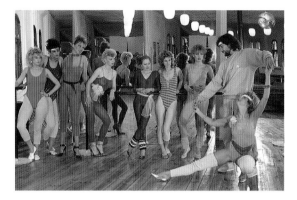

Hairy men were worshipped as gods in '80s gyms. Thanks to successful breeding programmes, they are now more commonplace, with less novelty value.

In the '80s, some premium gyms experimented with motivational dancing men in the weights area, but following what turned out to be chillingly well-founded health and safety concerns, they were withdrawn. Feel free to try this at home though.

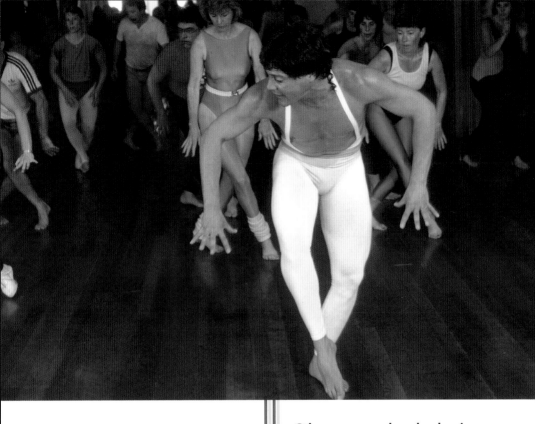

Other gyms employed a dancing man whose mantra was 'jazz hands are healthy hands'. This is as true today as it was then.

Don't let a lack of space prevent you from feeling the burn with your fitness-loving friends. Thanks to the slippery qualities of Lycra, you can squeeze hundreds of women into a local hotel restroom. Do not be discouraged if you look like members of a death cult.

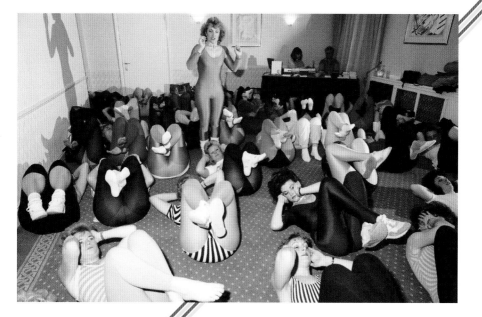

33

It's actually amazing how motivating
a swift kick to the head can be
when you're crammed into a
toddlers' swimming pool.

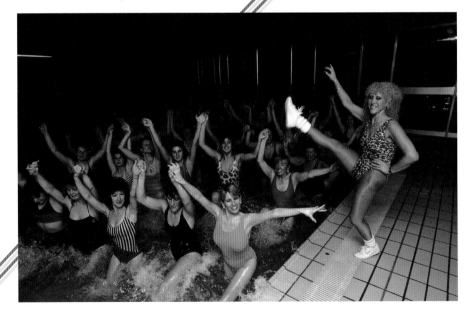

In the '80s, pools didn't have swimwear spinners, so adopting positions like this was the only way to accelerate the drying process. Incorporate this move into your daily laundry schedule and watch those wobbly thighs turn to steel.

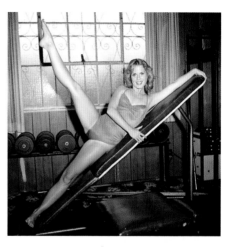

If today's outdoor boot camps are all a bit much, you might like to consider the popular '80s pursuit of *Mission Impossible*-style workouts. Taking place in luxurious settings, they involved crawling below invisible laser beams, but were discontinued due to the amount of static electricity they generated.

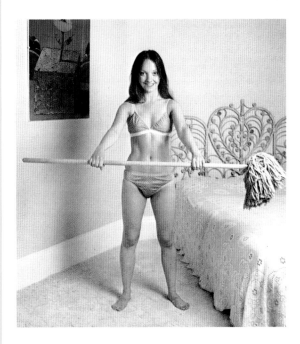

And finally, if you're too shy to work out in public, do it at home. Don't have the right equipment? Improvise. All you really need is a can-do attitude and some basic cleaning equipment.

LIVE IT

Like the powerfully musky scents favoured by the shoulder pad-wielding business ladies of the period, fitness culture permeated nearly every facet of '80s living.

Movies and music videos throbbed with the sight of gorgeous humans working their perfect physiques, while hard-bodied celebrities cashed in on the craze, releasing a never-ending stream of videos to show us civilians how to achieve those lean and glossy looks. It all looked like so much FUN.

So chuck those kale and avocado shakes and mindful exercise regimes on the fire, and throw yourself into the world of high-kicking, shoulder-revealing dramas, bizarre body-strengthening devices and other multi-coloured displays of gladiatorial excellence.

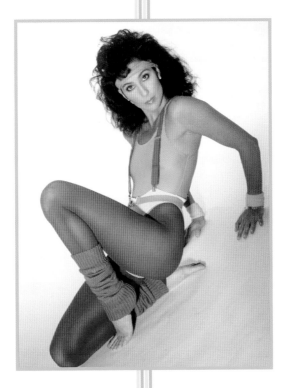

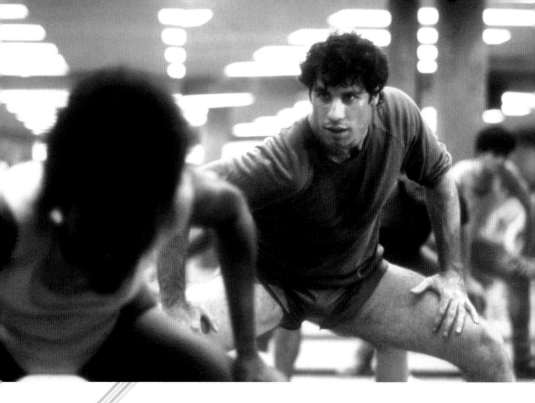

In the romantic '80s movie, *Perfect*, John Travolta played a reporter looking into the rise of health clubs as pick-up joints. It was all a valid excuse to show lean bodies in butt-creeping leotards, and pelvic thrusts formed an important part of the action.

...His co-star, Jamie Lee
Curtis, presents a solid case
as the love interest.

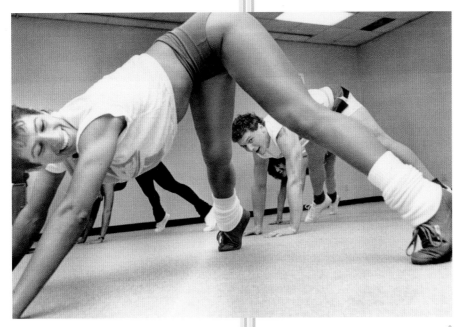

In the surprisingly dark film
Footloose, Kevin Bacon proved
that doing angry, balletic dancing
in your jeans was a sure-fire way
to affect radical societal change.

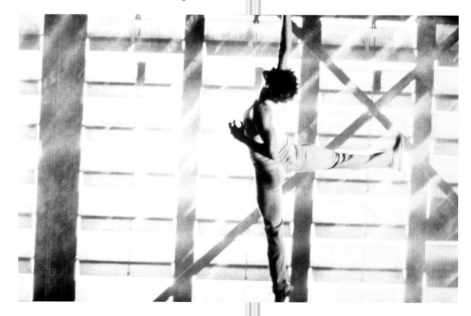

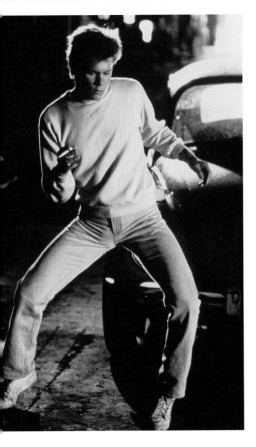

Doingdy-doingdy-doingdy-doing-doing. Dance away that oppression...

43

...And any other areas of concern.

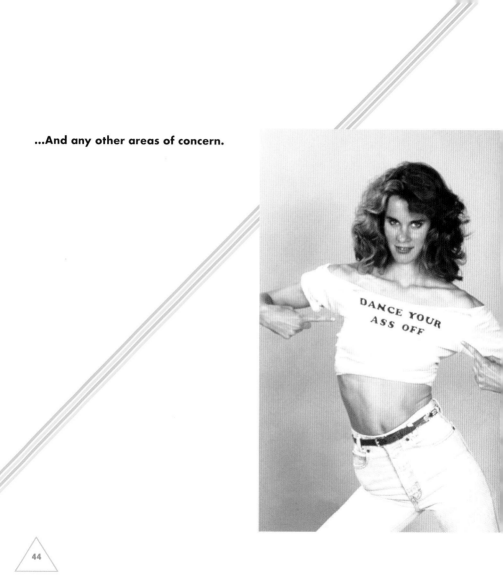

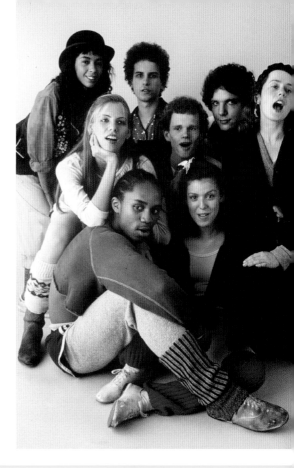

Fame, the movie about a bunch of ambitious stage-school kids, inspired a generation to sing and dance their little hearts out, stopping traffic with their talent...

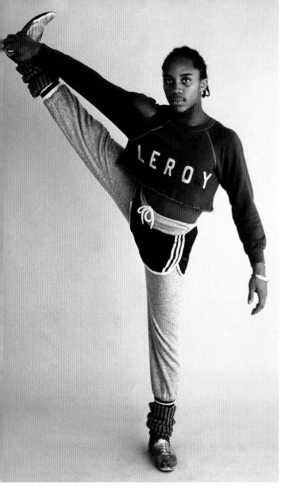

...And to wear shorts over their sweat pants – a style that's still popular among dancers hoping to disguise the fact that they've accidentally sat on a burrito.

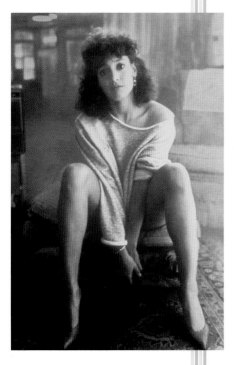

Flashdance taught us two of the most important life lessons: that a pretty shoulder peeping out of an oversized shirt is hella cute, and that you can be a welder by day and a dancer by night. Why the latter message isn't tattooed on more dreamers' lower backs is a mystery.

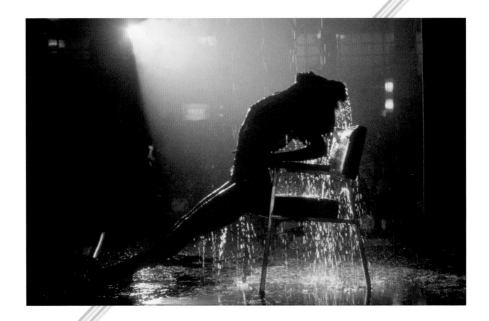

Unfortunately, in one scene Jennifer Beals's character freshens up on stage by flushing an invisible overhead lavatory – an act of gross irresponsibility. Any club manager worth their salt would have cordoned off the area immediately. If you must replicate this, please do it in the garden.

The formerly squeaky-clean Olivia Newton-John took a bold new direction in *Let's Get Physical,* a profound song exploring the ineffable ache of unrequited love and the Sisyphean pursuit of corporeal supremacy in a heteronormative culture. There's a subtle plot twist at the end of the raunchy video, though – the subject, no doubt, of hundreds of theses.

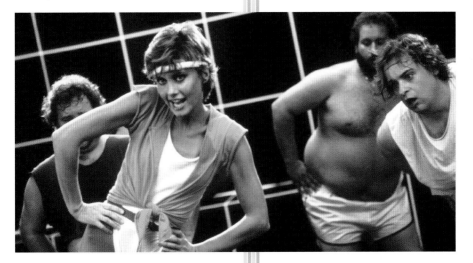

Usually when you see a man in the park wearing nothing but his jeans, holding what looks like a home-made crossbow, your instinct is to drop your belongings and RUN. But this was David Hasselhoff, and David Hasselhoff was famous, so nobody called the police.

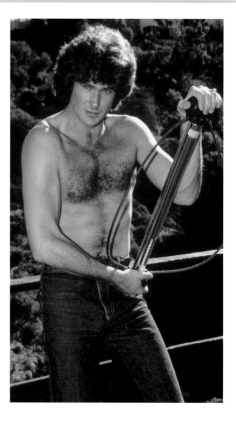

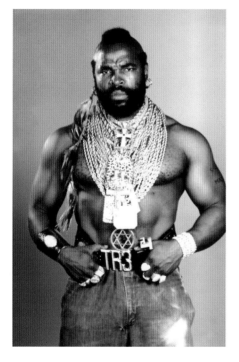

Mr T fell into the same denim trap as the Hoff, but distracted onlookers by showing off a unique new weight-lifting system, which involved integrating hernia-inducingly heavy jewellery into his daily life.

Mr Motivator was such a bouncy presence on British screens that people thought their televisions were faulty. We never did find out what was in that bumbag.

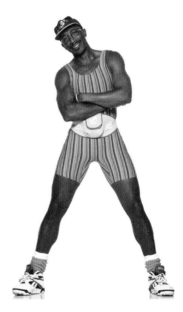

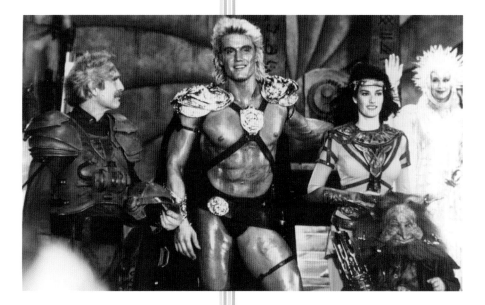

Hollywood couldn't get enough of muscle men in the '80s. Former martial artist Dolph Lundgren, pictured here in *Masters of the Universe,* may have received some unkind reviews for his acting, but his gift to the world was being able to make every single person who stood next to him feel like the poor fellow on the bottom right.

If you're still attached to your cuddly toys, take a leaf out of Joanna Lumley's book and work out with a despondent, flaccid-bodied Pink Panther.

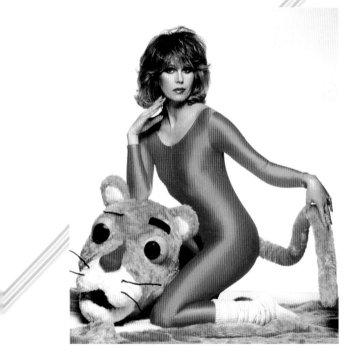

Add an element of danger to your chest-firming workout, as Charlie's Angel Jaclyn Smith did, by selecting a product able to nip and yank even the shortest of body hairs.

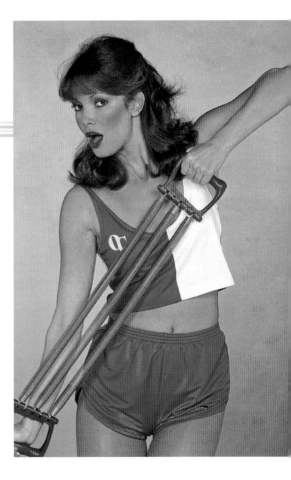

While burning calories with style was a big part of the '80s, people were also learning about how to consume them cleverly. Uptown girl Christie Brinkley proved that you could avert your cravings for sugar by dressing from head to toe in colours sweet enough to make your teeth hurt.

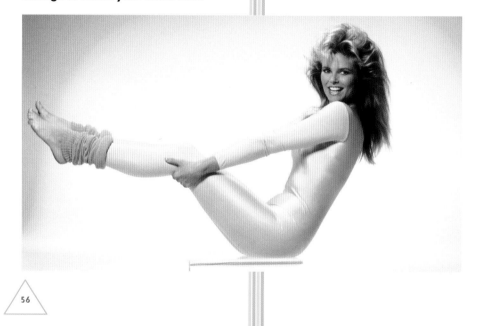

Sugar-free drinks did really well in countries where the brand name wasn't local slang for 'cigarette'.

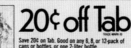

Body
by Tab.

Jayne Kennedy

20¢ off Tab

Save 20¢ on Tab. Good on any 6, 8, or 12-pack of cans or bottles, or one 2-liter bottle.

NOTE TO DEALER: For each coupon you accept as our authorized agent, we will pay you the face value of this coupon, plus 7¢ handling charges, provided you and your customers have complied with the terms of this offer. Any other application constitutes fraud. Invoices showing your purchase of sufficient stock to cover all coupons must be shown upon request. Void where prohibited, taxed or restricted. Your customer must pay any required sales tax and bottle deposit. Cash value 1/20 of 1¢. Redeem by mailing to: The Coca-Cola Company, PO Box 1504, Clinton, Iowa 52734.

LIMIT: ONE COUPON PER PURCHASE. OFFER EXPIRES DECEMBER 31, 1983. "TAB" is a registered trade-mark of The Coca-Cola Company.
© 1983 The Coca-Cola Company.

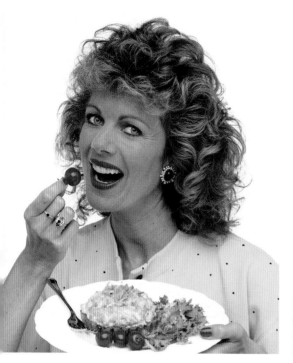

British fitness guru Lizzie Webb showed us that being perpetually about to eat delicious food was much more slimming than actually eating it.

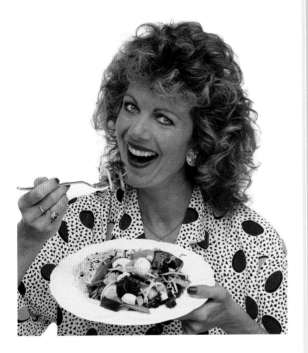

...And that changing your outfit
between courses could distract
you from the hunger.

No amount of wordplay, alas,
could detract from the fact that this
appetite-supressing product had
a genuinely unfortunate name.

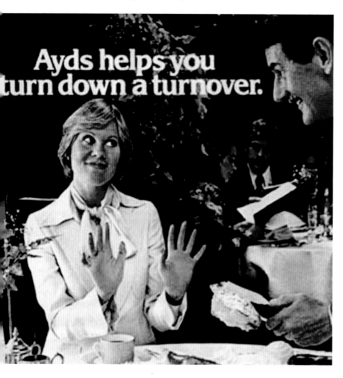

It's almost as if Cher saw
that one coming.

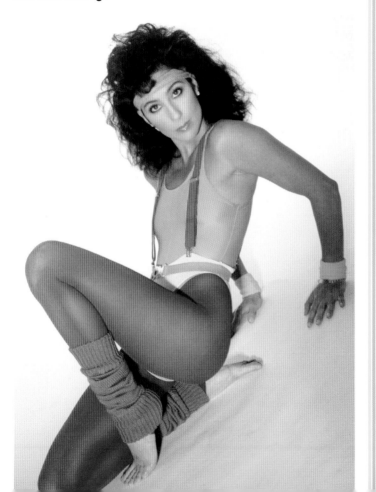

Jane Fonda was the undisputed queen of the workout video. Formerly known as 'Hanoi Jane' due to her opposition to the war in Vietnam, her public promotion of the body beautiful helped her ditch her political baggage as quickly as her devotees shed excess pounds.

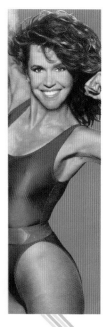

FOLLOW THE LEADER.

Jane Fonda, naturally. Now join the millions of active women who work out with her every day. With Jane Fonda's new COMPLETE WORKOUT video you've got it all—the aerobics, conditioning and stretching routines that you combine to match your own fitness level and personal goals. From the 70-minute "whole-body" workout to shorter routines for spot toning and shaping, create a program that suits your busy day. And let Jane Fonda's COMPLETE WORKOUT lead you through a New Year of feeling better and looking healthier than ever before!

Jane Fonda's COMPLETE WORKOUT. Now in video stores everywhere.

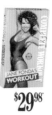

29^{98*}

Now on
videocassette.

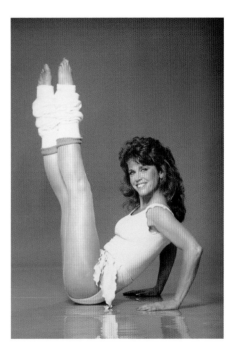

...And she inadvertently discovered an attractive new way to help people get rid of trapped wind. On behalf of over-eaters the world over, we thank you, Jane.

Side A

1 *Gonna Fly Now / Rocky's Theme*

2 *Go For It All*

3 *Stronger Every Day*

Side B

1 *I Love My Bike*

2 *Sit-Up-Wrap*

3 *Gonna Fly Now / Rocky's Theme (reprise)*

The chunky fellows got in on the act too. Sylvester Stallone's *Rocky Fun and Fitness* workout presumably did not include chasing a chicken down a grotty back street or being beaten to a pulp in front of a braying crowd while your wife cried beside the ring.

ROCKY

Fun
and
Fitness

FREE ROCKY
EXERCISE POSTER
INCLUDED

Kid
Stuff
RECORDS & TAPES

KSB 1018

Arnold Schwarzenegger's Total Body Workout

Side A

Without Weights

1 Gladys Knight & The Pips – *Save The Overtime For Me*

2 Journey – *Don't Stop Believin'*

3 Tommy Tutone – *867-5309 (Jenny)*

4 Champaign – *Let Your Body Rock*

5 Michael Case Kissel – *Love Not War*

6 Eddie Money – *Think I'm In Love*

7 Deniece Williams – *I'm So Proud*

Side B

With Weights

1 Gladys Knight & The Pips – *Save The Overtime For Me*

2 The Weather Girls – *It's Raining Men*

3 Champaign – *Let Your Body Rock*

4 Michael Case Kissel – *Love Not War*

5 Blue Öyster Cult – *Burning For You*

6 Deniece Williams – *I'm So Proud*

Arnold Schwarzenegger's Total Body Workout carried some tantalisingly camp tracks, including It's Raining Men by The Weather Girls. Perhaps you'd like to sing that – loudly – in Arnie's accent next time you're pumping iron.

Side A
1 *Aerobics Boogie*
2 *High Intensity*
3 *Release*
4 *Mellow Moments*
Side B
1 *Movin' Fever*
2 *Pizazz*
3 *Relaxation*

Workout albums became increasingly specialised in the '80s. You could even get records that helped you focus on one particular body part, often presented by sisters who could only bend one leg.

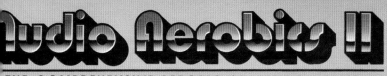

Audio Aerobics II

THE COMPREHENSIVE AEROBIC CLASSROOM SERIES

WAIST & STOMACH!

PROFESSIONAL INSTRUCTORS: LESLIE & STACY LILIEN

ILLUSTRATED GUIDEBOOK INCLUDED

planta
Reco
PLP ★
STER

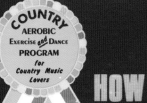

COUNTRY
AEROBIC
EXERCISE and DANCE
PROGRAM
for
Country Music
Lovers

HOW THE *Waist* WAS WON

"THE COUNTRY WAY FROM TRUE GRIT TO TRUE FIT"

June LaSalvia

FREE
COMPLETE ILLUSTRATED
INSTRUCTION POSTER PLUS
WEIGHT REDUCTION SUGGESTIONS
FIT • AS / A • FIDDLE • COUNTRY
TUNE-UP / SHAPE-UP EXERCISES
FOR THE ENTIRE FAMILY

*Featuring
The Hits...*

9 TO 5
ELVIRA
ROCKY TOP
TULSA TIME
Plus Others

Side A

1 *Get Up Off Your Good Intentions*
2 *Tulsa Time*
3 *Nine To Five*
4 *Rocky Top*
5 *I Love To Dance*

Side B

1 *Elvira*
2 *Before The Next Teardrop Falls*
3 *Turn The World Around The Other Way*
4 *Intro To Relaxation*
5 *Daydream*

Weak puns became as important as hard buns, and albums started targeting people according to their musical and aesthetic tastes. In this one, headbands and leg warmers were swapped for Stetsons and cowgirl boots as punters were encouraged to go from 'true grit to true fit'. Why not bring a bedazzled saddle to your next spin class? Ride on, rhinestone cowgirl!

Side A
1 *Sensuous Warm-Ups*
2 *Pelvic Pleasures*
3 *Lover's Lunge*
4 *Turn & Tease Me*
5 *Stripper's Strut*
6 *Rotations For Arousal*
Side B
1 *Body Manipulations*
2 *Kinky Chorus Kick & Flash*
3 *The Shameless Shake*
4 *The Fan Dance*
5 *Sexy Suzy*
6 *Curl His Toes Curl-Ups*

Erotic Aerobics? I mean, what other kind is there?

EROTIC AEROBICS

Sensuous exercises to improve your love life! Featuring easy-to-follow visual & vocal instructions.

This unique package contains both a Record and a Cassette for twice the listening pleasure.

Ronco™

A Ron Harris Presentation

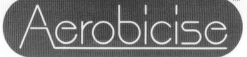

Aerobicise™

The California Exercise Craze

AS SEEN ON

Side A
Class one
1 *Bella Bella*
2 *Ajitto*
3 *One Hand Clapping*
3 *I'm Only Human*
4 *Skin*
Class two
1 *One More Way*
2 *Flat Out*
3 *Go For It*
8 *Sweet N' Nasty*
Side B
Class three
1 *Show Me*
2 *What Does It Take*
3 *Hot Sox*
4 *Ode To Joy*
5 *Hit It*
6 *Never Gonna Give You Up*

Inject some '80s rrrrrroooar
into your regime by channelling
your inner lioness.

75

Side A

1 Denny Correll – *Living Water*

2 The Mighty Clouds Of Joy – *Jesus Is The Rock*

3 Al Green – *Hallelujah (I Just Want To Praise The Lord)*

4 Imperials – *Stand By The Power*

5 Leon Patillo – *Saved*

Side B

1 B.J. Thomas – *The Unclouded Day*

2a Morris Chapman – *Longtime Friends*

2b Imperials – *I'm Forgiven*

3 Al Green – *His Name Is Jesus*

4 Dion – *Hearts Made Of Stone*

5 Amy Grant – *El Shaddai*

The '80s were the golden age of exercise programmes featuring Christian music. If you don't have anyone to spot you, perhaps you might like to stretch for our saviour.

A Complete Exercise Program Featuring Today's Finest Christian Music

Firm Believer®

cludes
lly illustrated
struction
ooklet

Featuring the music of:
IMPERIALS
AMY GRANT
AL GREEN
B.J. THOMAS
LEON PATILLO
DION
MIGHTY CLOUDS OF JOY
MORRIS CHAPMAN
DENNY CORRELL

Choreographed Exercise to Contemporary Gospel Music

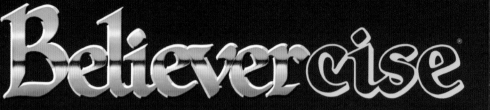

Believercise

DaySpring

Illustrated instruction poster included

Side A
1 B.J. Thomas – *Without A Doubt*
2 The Happy Goodman Family – *Only The Sound Of His Trumpet*
3 Amy Grant – *I Have Decided*
4 Leon Patillo – *Dance Children Dance*
5 Imperials – *Any Good Time At All*
Side B
1 Amy Grant – *In A Little While*
2 Benny Hester – *Nobody Knows Me Like You (Edited Version)*
3 The Happy Goodman Family – *He Walked Upon The Water*
4 Leon Patillo – *Don't Give In*
5 The Gaither Vocal Band – *I'm Yours*
6 Imperials – *Because Of Who You Are*

Justin Bieber fans might like to adapt and incorporate this powerful pun into their own routines.

Side A

1 Clarence Williams, Thomas Waller – *Squeeze Me*

2 Norman Whitfield – *Which Way Is Up*

3 Mike Post, Pete Carpenter – *Rockford Files*

4 Don Ray, Hughie Prince – *Boogie Woogie Bugle Boy*

5 Stephen Bishop – *Animal House*

6 Gene DePaul, Sammy Cahn – *Teach Me Tonight*

Side B

1 Dave Grusin, Morgan Ames – *Baretta's Theme*

2 Ronnie Self – *Sweet Nothin's*

3 Norman Whitfield – *Car Wash*

4 Everett Robbins, Porter Grainger – *T'aint Nobody's Biz-ness If I Do*

5 Antonio Carlos Jobim – *Girl From Ipanema*

6 Brian Potter, Dennis Lambert – *Don't Pull Your Love*

Ah, Jazzercise – proof that real style never goes out of fashion.

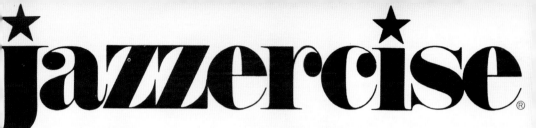

jazzercise

By Judi Sheppard Missett

The jazz-dance fitness program that conditions your body, lifts your spirit, puts a smile on your face and a bounce in your step!

A WILD AND WOOLLY WORKOUT!

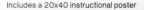

Includes a 20x40 instructional poster

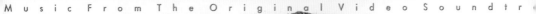

Music From The Original Video Soundtra

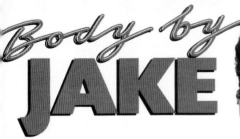

DON'T
QUIT

JAKE

Side A
1 *Don't Quit*
2 *Hard Work*
3 *Baby Work Out*
4 *Pump It Up*
Side B
1 *Toughen Up*
2 *You Can Get It If You Really Want*
3 *Hard As A Rock*
4 *Firepower*

Jake won't let you quit. He won't get lost either because it says 'Jake' on his belt.

Companies trying to help people take health and fitness shortcuts did a roaring trade in the '80s. This one made a virtue of the fact that it looked like an Ikea chaise lounge tearfully abandoned halfway through construction.

Can you find the muscle building machine in this picture?

People even started incorporating their pets into their workouts, though it is believed this was more to do with needing them as smell decoys in hot rooms filled with synthetic fibre–generated sweat.

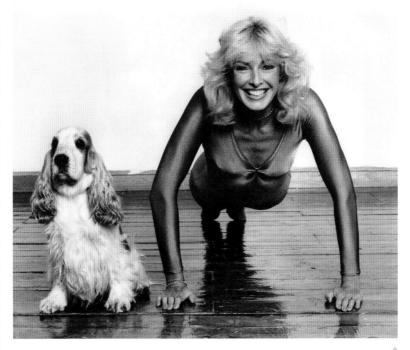

And as the price of designer workout wear sky-rocketed, competition became fierce, which took its toll on friendships. On the plus side, this inspired the birth of gladiatorial game shows – a joyful new way of twisting your ankle on national television.

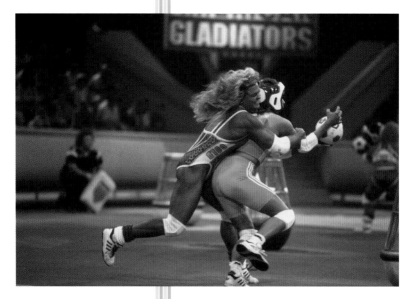

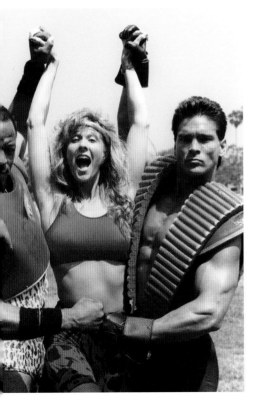

The sudden surplus of personal trainers meant that many women were now able to afford to pay two men to help with their stretching. Why not try making new friends in the gym by asking them to help you with your lats?

FLAUNT IT

What's the point of putting in all that time and work at the gym if you're not going to show off the results? You've done the pain part – now it's time to indulge in those gains.

The '80s were all about standing out from the crowd, and this was achieved through a complicated process of asset embellishment. Anyone who left more than 20 per cent of their body's surface area unadorned ran the very real risk of not being noticed, which, back then, was worse than actual death.

So take inspiration from the neon age of posing and work it. Work it hard. And repeat after me: it's what's on the outside that counts!

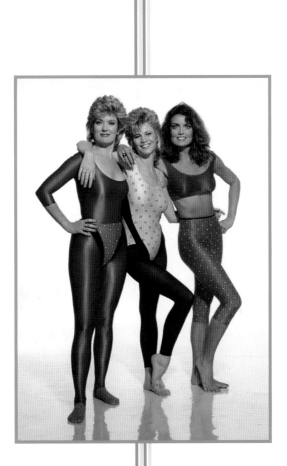

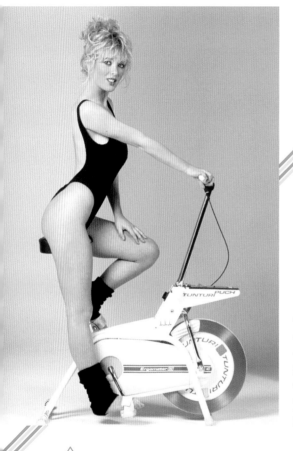

The first thing to remember is that you don't actually have to exercise when you go the gym, especially if the cut of your leotard is making you feel shy. Simply arrange yourself on a piece of equipment and practise your facial expressions.

If there's a ladder at your exercise club, that's even better. Nothing says 'come hither, for I am as upwardly mobile as I am fit' like perching on a piece of building equipment. In heels.

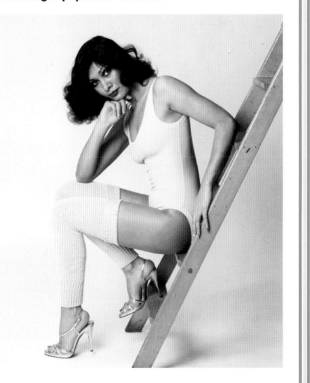

Consider improvising with an ironing board if all the equipment is taken. This way you can send out subtle signals that as well as being a cast-iron stunner, you'd be useful around the house too.

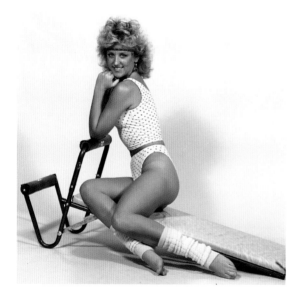

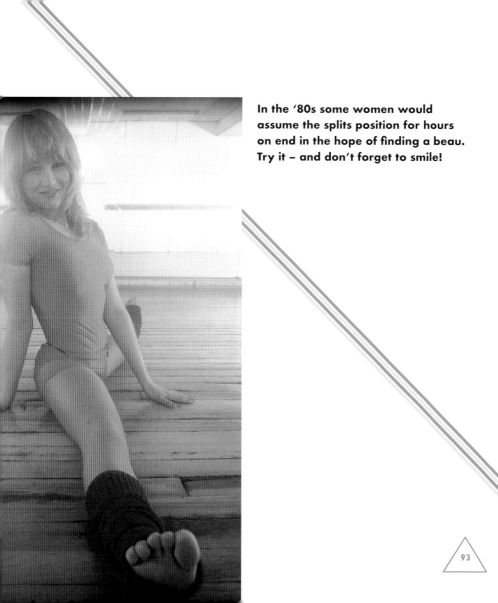

In the '80s some women would assume the splits position for hours on end in the hope of finding a beau. Try it – and don't forget to smile!

Smile to hide the cramp in your foot.

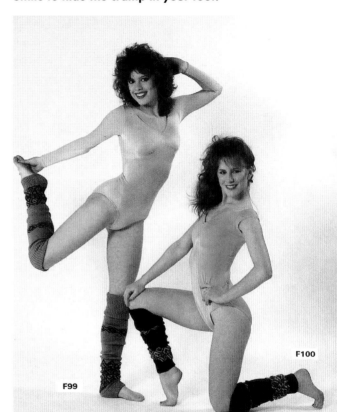

F99

F100

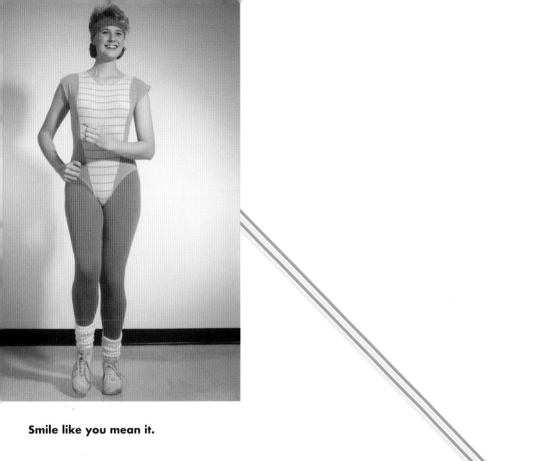

Smile like you mean it.

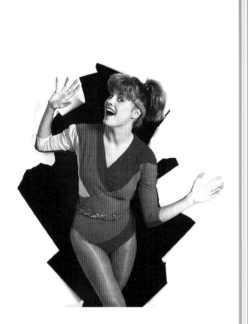

Seriously, smile as if your
very life depends on it.

Or don't. Sultry's an awesome look
too. You've totally earned it, girl.

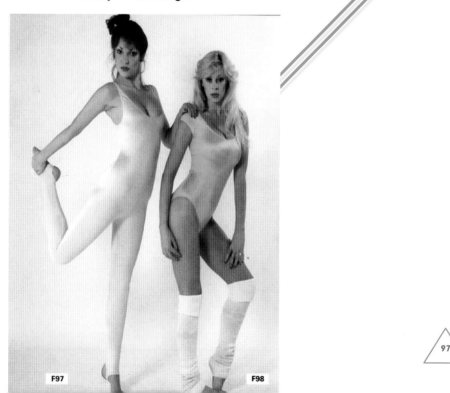

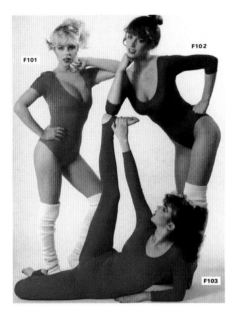

F101

F102

F103

When you're trying to show off your lean thighs but want to look casual about it, try this hack: pop your elbow on your friend's heel like it's no big thing.

I mean, it's not a competition
or anything.

Just a bit of friendly rivalry.

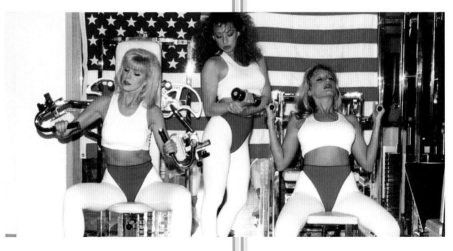

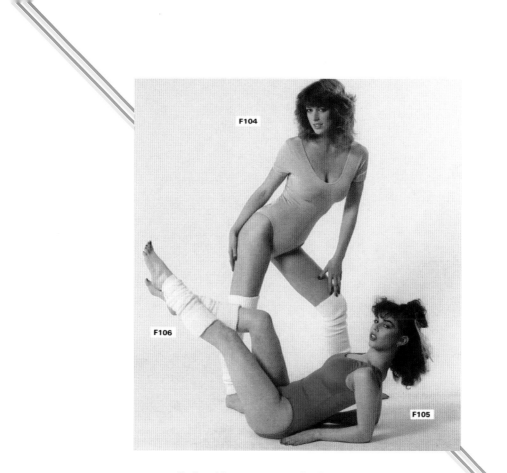

It's totally healthy to want to look
hotter than your frenemies.

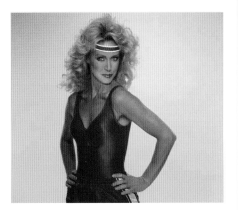

To the victor, the matching headband!

Feel free to celebrate your physical superiority in whatever way you see fit. This is YOUR time. Own that glory.

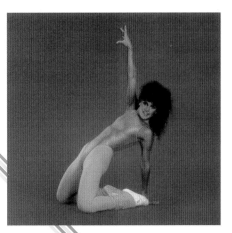

Leotards were cut super-high round the thighs in the '80s, coinciding with a peak in the deployment of animal prints. This caused a perfect storm of flauntwear...

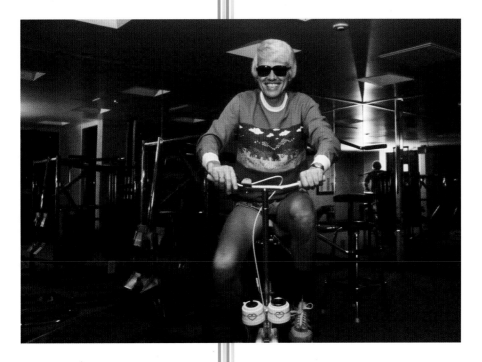

...which meant a lot of fellow gym-goers found happiness they'd never dreamt possible but didn't always know where to look.

Roller-skating really took off in the '80s. As well as being an environmentally friendly form of getting from A to B, it was a perfect way of ensuring you'd displayed your bodywork to the widest possible audience.

I mean, who can resist the combination of skates, leg warmers AND a headband?

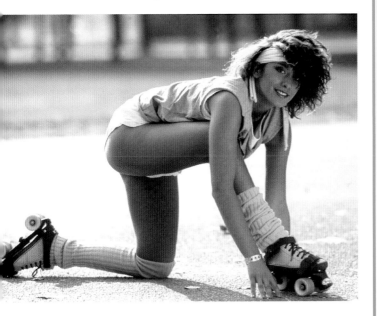

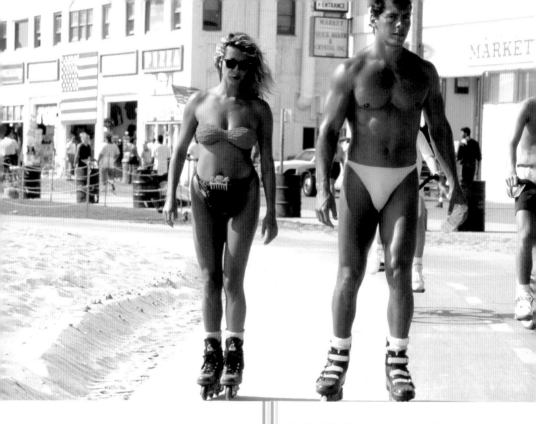

Rollerblading was pretty hot in the '80s too. Blend those wheels with fluorescent swimwear and a rock-hard, tanned body for maximum impact. Just don't fall – imagine the road rash...

But even if you don't have the self-confidence, or indeed balance, to take your show on the road, you've gotta keep telling yourself how amazing you are. Fake it till you make it.

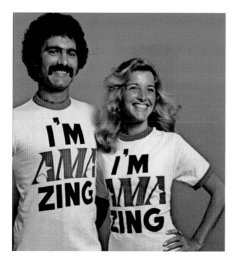

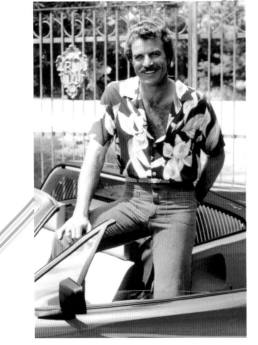

And never, I say NEVER, deprive the world of that hot bod of yours. Guys, make like Magnum and invest in a Hawaiian shirt to show off your furry chest, then perch your steely buns on a sports car. Doesn't matter if it's not yours.

Butts were huge in the '80s, not in
the same way they are now though.
Double denim – double trouble.
Or quadruple, in this instance.

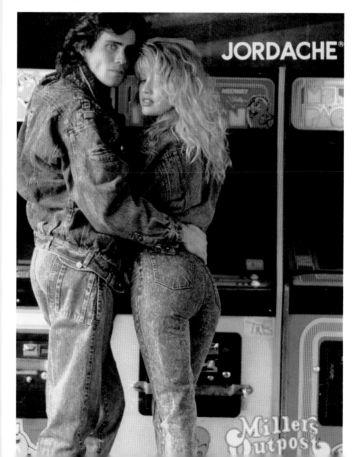

You've worked for that butt –
now hitch a topless ride off your
boyfriend to ensure everyone
appreciates your glute work.

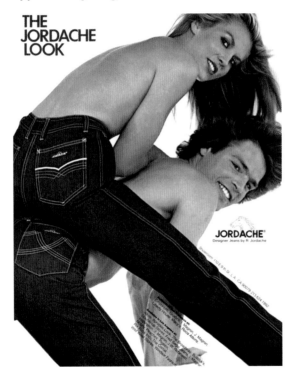

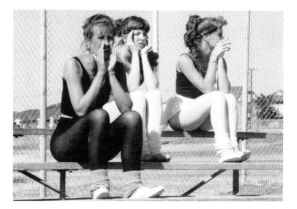

Pretending to support somebody else's sporting endeavours while wearing aerobics gear was a big part of '80s life. Bring the concept up to date by wearing yoga pants to spy on your boyfriend while he plays computer games.

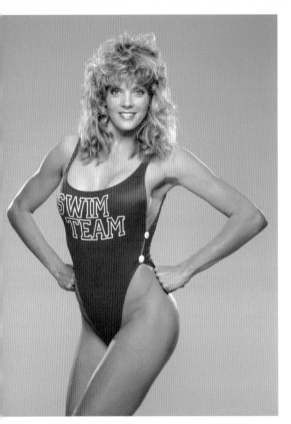

Poolside posing is art. Practise
by only ever breathing in.

If you've been inspired by athlete Florence Griffith-Joiner – AKA Flo-Jo – to grow your nails super-long, beware: those talons go through leggings like a hot knife through hair mousse, and you might end up with one bare leg.

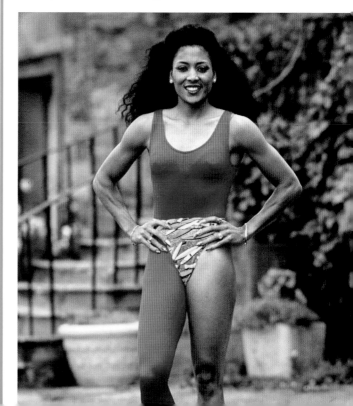

As people developed more body confidence in the '80s, aerobics started being enjoyed beyond the gym and evolved into more of a performance, occasionally looking like a flashmob in a maximum-security prison.

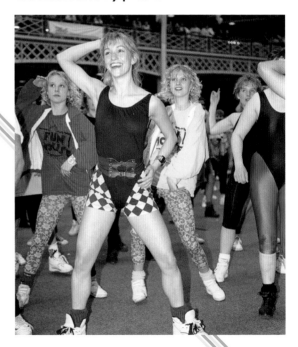

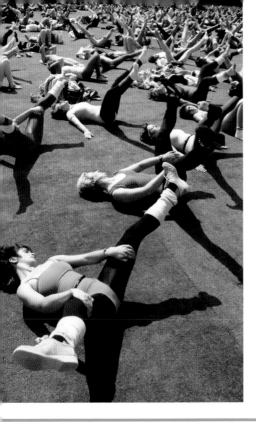

Football pitches throughout the world became jam-packed with people who looked like they were offering unconventional salutations to the sun god.

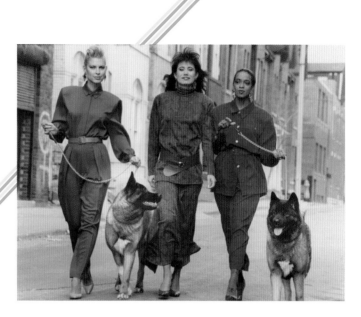

Unfortunately, few among us will ever achieve the level of panache '80s ladies had (in part because shoulder pads the size of surf boards are so hard to come by these days), but we all need something to aim for.

So get out there, and get physical! And whatever form of exercise you choose, the main thing to remember is to reach for the sky, and do it with enthusiasm! Or just wear your underpants on the outside – it's a start...

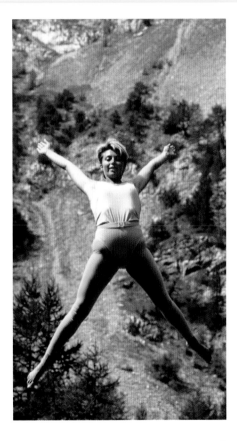

PHOTOGRAPHY CREDITS

To the fearless (and shameless) women and men who grace these pages, thank you for embodying all that is excellent about the fittest decade of them all. We who are about to work out salute you.

Best efforts have been made to trace the original copyright holders of the images included in this collection. The publishers will be pleased to make good any omissions or rectify any mistakes brought to their attention at the earliest opportunity.

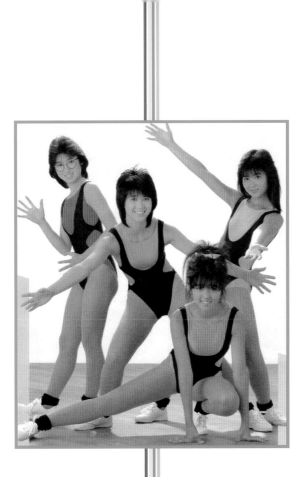

Page 2: ©Martin Lawrence / Associated
  Newspapers / REX / Shutterstock
Page 7: ©Harry Langdon / Getty Images

Chapter 1: Work It
Page 9: ©Directphoto Collection
  / Alamy Stock Photo
Page 10: ©Universal Images Group North
  America LLC / Alamy Stock Photo
Page 11: With thanks to scanagogo.com
Page 12: With thanks to scanagogo.com
Page 13: ©Benjamin Auger / Paris
  Match via Getty Images
Page 14: ©Norman Mosallem
  / REX / Shutterstock
Page 15: ©Globe Photos Inc
  / REX / Shutterstock
Page 16: ©ARCHIVE PHOTOS
  / REX / Shutterstock
Page 17: ©Mike Forster / Associated
  Newspapers / REX / Shutterstock
Page 18: With thanks to scanagogo.com
Page 19: ©Directphoto Collection
  / Alamy Stock Photo

Page 20: ©George Tiedemann / The LIFE
  Images Collection / Getty Images
Page 21: With thanks to scanagogo.com
Page 22: With thanks to scanagogo.com
Page 23: With thanks to scanagogo.com
Page 24: ©Slimming Magazine
  / REX / Shutterstock
Page 25: ©SLIMMING MAGAZINE
  / REX / Shutterstock
Page 26: ©Matsumoto / AP
  / REX / Shutterstock
Page 27: With thanks to scanagogo.com
Page 28: With thanks to scanagogo.com
Page 29: ©Joan Adlen / Getty Images
Page 30: With thanks to scanagogo.com
Page 31: ©Sipa Press / REX / Shutterstock
Page 32: ©Matthew Naythons / The LIFE
  Images Collection / Getty Images
Page 33: ©Mirrorpix / Doreen Spooner
Page 34: ©Ian Turner / REX / Shutterstock
Page 35: With thanks to scanagogo.com
Page 36: ©Manuel Litran/Paris
  Match via Getty Images
Page 37: With thanks to scanagogo.com

Chapter 2: Live It

Page 39: ©Harry Langdon / Getty Images
Page 40: ©Photo 12 / Alamy Stock Photo
Page 41: ©David Cooper / Toronto
 Star via Getty Images
Page 42: ©Paramount / Kobal
 / REX / Shutterstock
Page 43: ©Paramount / Kobal
 / REX / Shutterstock
Page 44: ©Paramount / Kobal
 / REX / Shutterstock
Page 45: ©MGM / Kobal
 / REX / Shutterstock
Page 46: ©MGM / Kobal /
 REX / Shutterstock
Page 47: ©Moviestore Collection
 / REX / Shutterstock
Page 48: ©Everett Collection
 Inc / Alamy Stock Photo
Page 49: ©Michael Ochs
 Archives / Getty Images
Page 50: ©FOTOS INTERNATIONAL
 / REX / Shutterstock
Page 51: ©Moviestore Collection
 / REX / Shutterstock

Page 52: ©ITV / REX / Shutterstock
Page 53: ©Moviestore collection
 Ltd / Alamy Stock Photo
Page 54: ©REX / Shutterstock
Page 55: With thanks to scanagogo.com
Page 56: ©Bettmann / Contributor
 / Getty Images
Page 57: Image courtesy of The
 Advertising Archives
Page 58: ©Victor Watts / REX / Shutterstock
Page 59: ©Victor Watts / REX / Shutterstock
Page 60: Image courtesy of The
 Advertising Archives
Page 61: ©Harry Langdon / Getty Images
Page 62: Image courtesy of The
 Advertising Archives
Page 63: ©Harry Langdon / Getty Images
Page 65: ©Kid Stuff Records. Image
 courtesy of Jive Time Records,
 Seattle; jivetimerecords.com
Page 66: ©Columbia Records. Image
 courtesy of Jive Time Records,
 Seattle; jivetimerecords.com

ACKNOWLEDGEMENTS

Thank you to *Desperately Seeking Susan*-era Madonna, who taught us grateful daughters of the '80s how to combine backcombed hair, slutty makeup and excessive jewellery with swaggering, dance-led athleticism. We had a ball. A sweaty, sweaty ball.

ABOUT THE AUTHOR

Ashley Davies is a journalist, columnist and advertising copywriter whose work has appeared in several publications, including *The Scotsman, The Guardian, The Times* and *Standard Issue*. She also runs the animal humour site, The Lab Report.

At the age of 13, she fashioned her first pair of leg warmers out of her dad's socks, and spent the 1980s indulging in some of the most atrocious fashions of the period, from crispy yellow perms and blue eyeshadow to dangerously tanned skin and flashes of neon. She has since come to realise there are other ways to get attention.

She lives in the seaside town of North Berwick, near Edinburgh in Scotland. She likes gawping at animals.

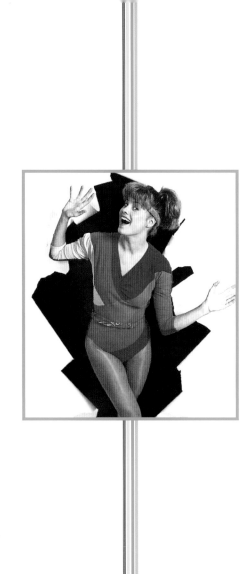